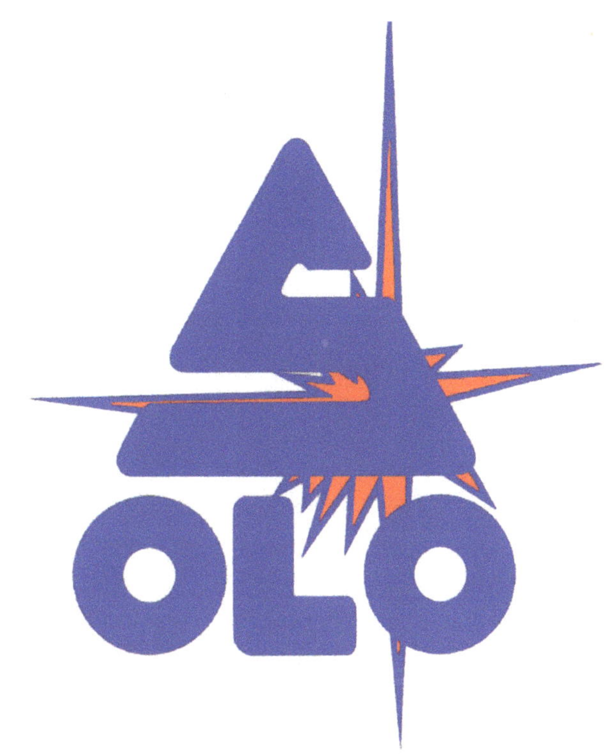

SOLO Cardiopulmonary Resuscitation (CPR)

SOLO 心肺蘇生法 (CPR)

English/Japanese Edition
Translated by Naomi O'Keeffe
and Daisuke Kondo

Our work, teaching, and materials is gratefully dedicated to all those who generously give of their time, care, compassion, and expertise to help those in need regardless of race, age, sex, nationality, or ethnicity. With all our thanks, SOLO
私達が行っている業務、教育、また使用している教材は、人種、年齢、性別、国籍、民族に関係なく、困っている人を助ける為に、自分の時間、ケア、思いやり、また専門知識を惜しみなく与える全ての方の為に提供しております。心より感謝致します。SOLOより

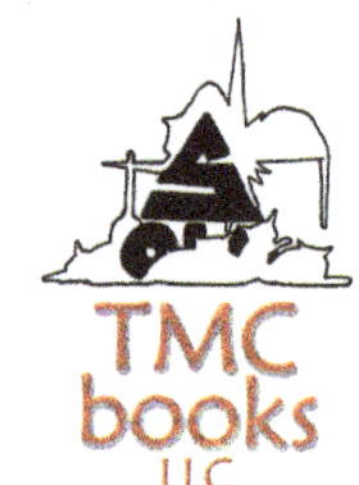

TMC BOOKS LLC
731 Tasker Hill Rd,
Conway, NH 03818
USA
www.tmcbooks.com

THE HEART
心臓

AORTA 大動脈
PULMONARY ARTERY 肺動脈
LEFT ATRIUM 左心房
右心房 RIGHT ATRIUM
LEFT ANTERIOR 左冠動脈前下行枝
DESCENDING （左冠状動脈）
ARTERY
(CORONARY
ARTERY)
右冠状動脈 RIGHT CORONARY ARTERY
LEFT VENTRICLE 左心室
右心室 RIGHT VENTRICLE

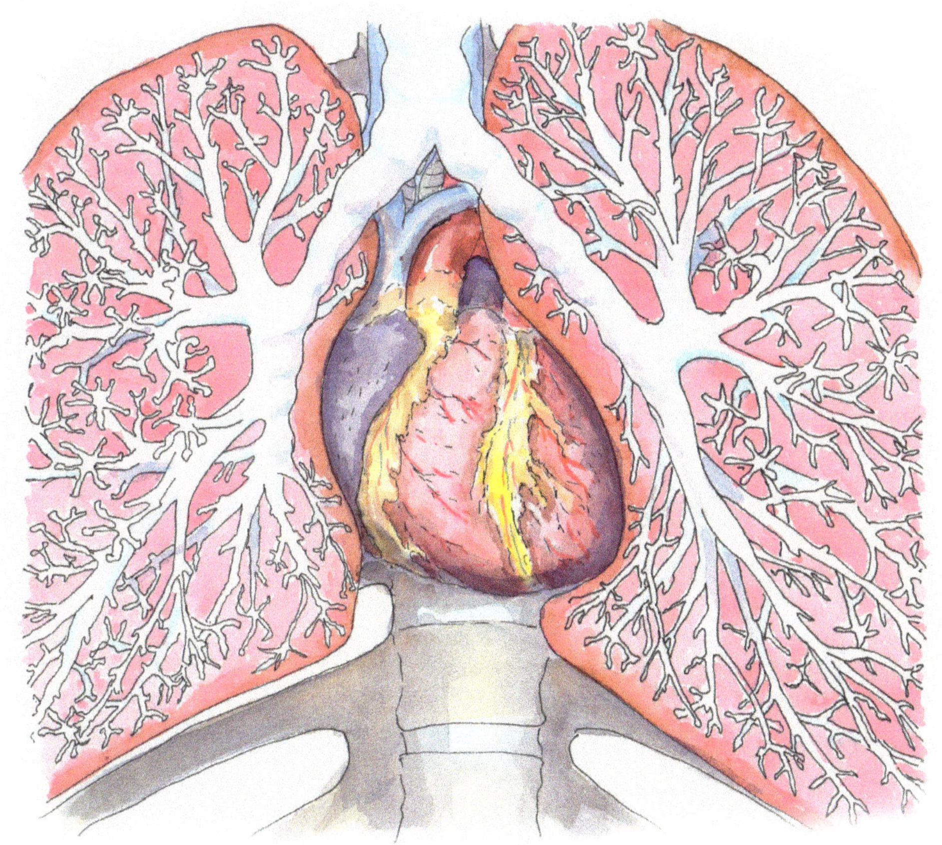

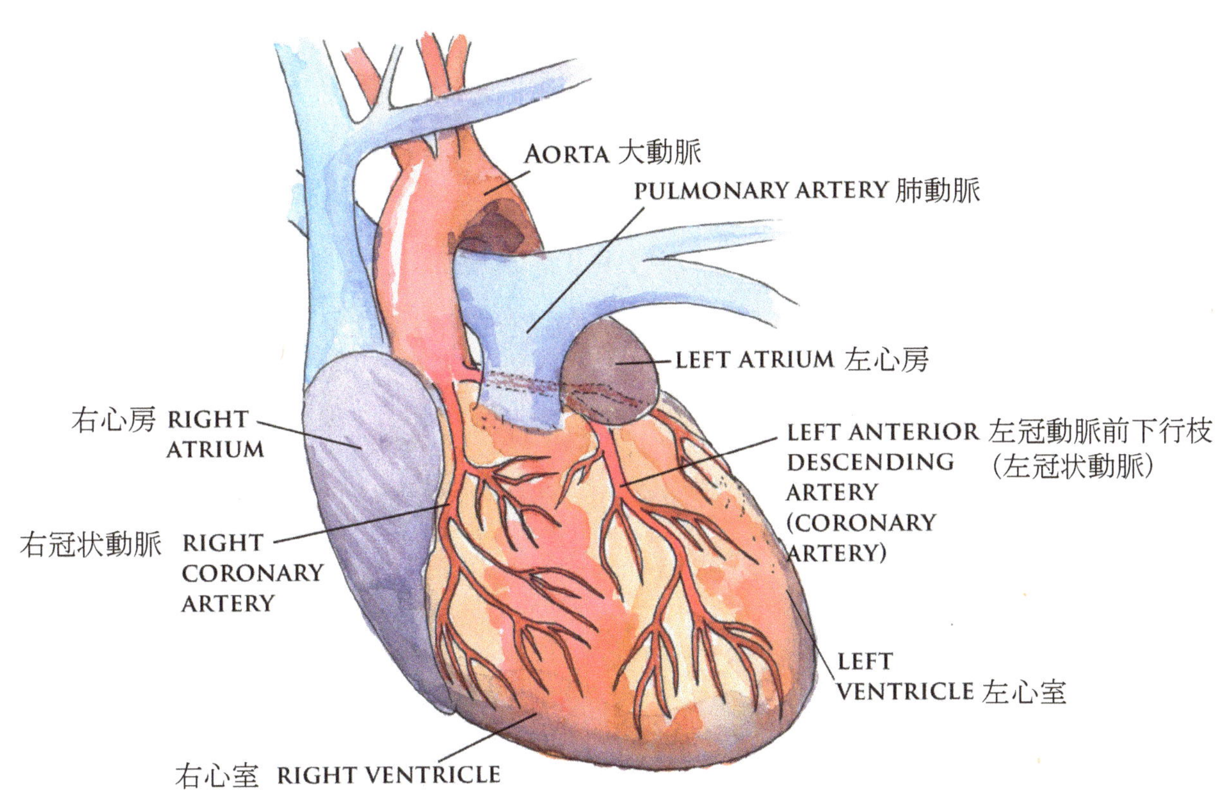

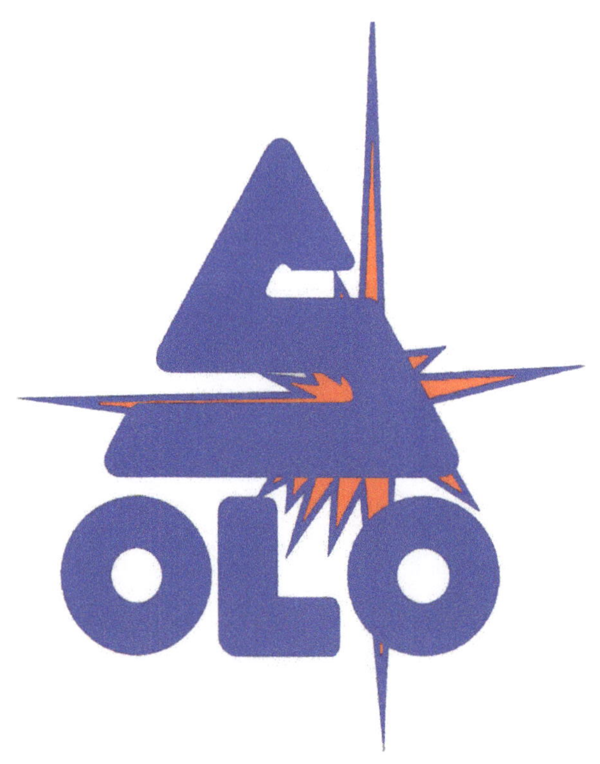

SOLO Cardiopulmonary Resuscitation (CPR)

SOLO 心肺蘇生法 (CPR)

English/Japanese Edition
Translated by Naomi O'Keeffe
and Daisuke Kondo

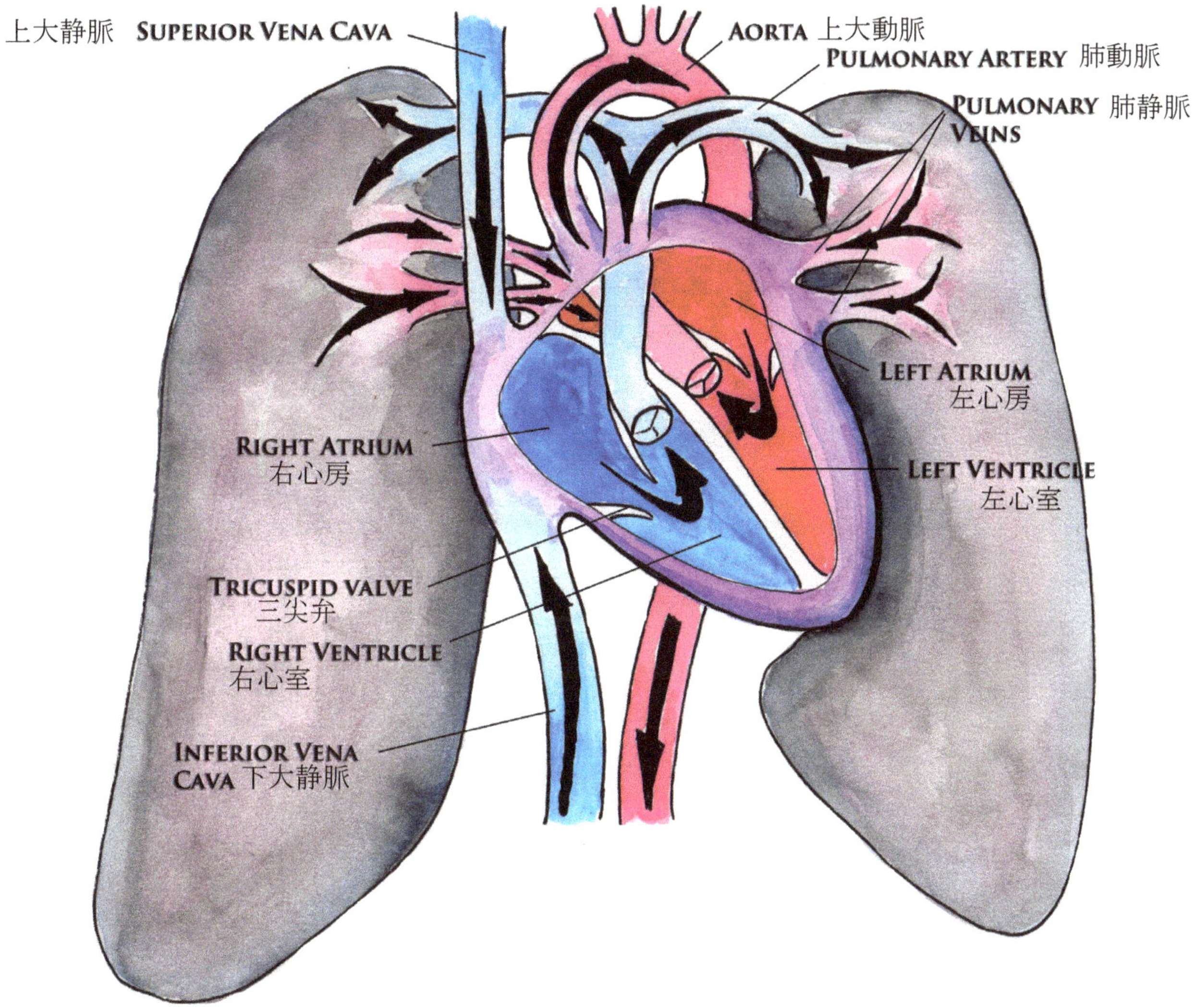

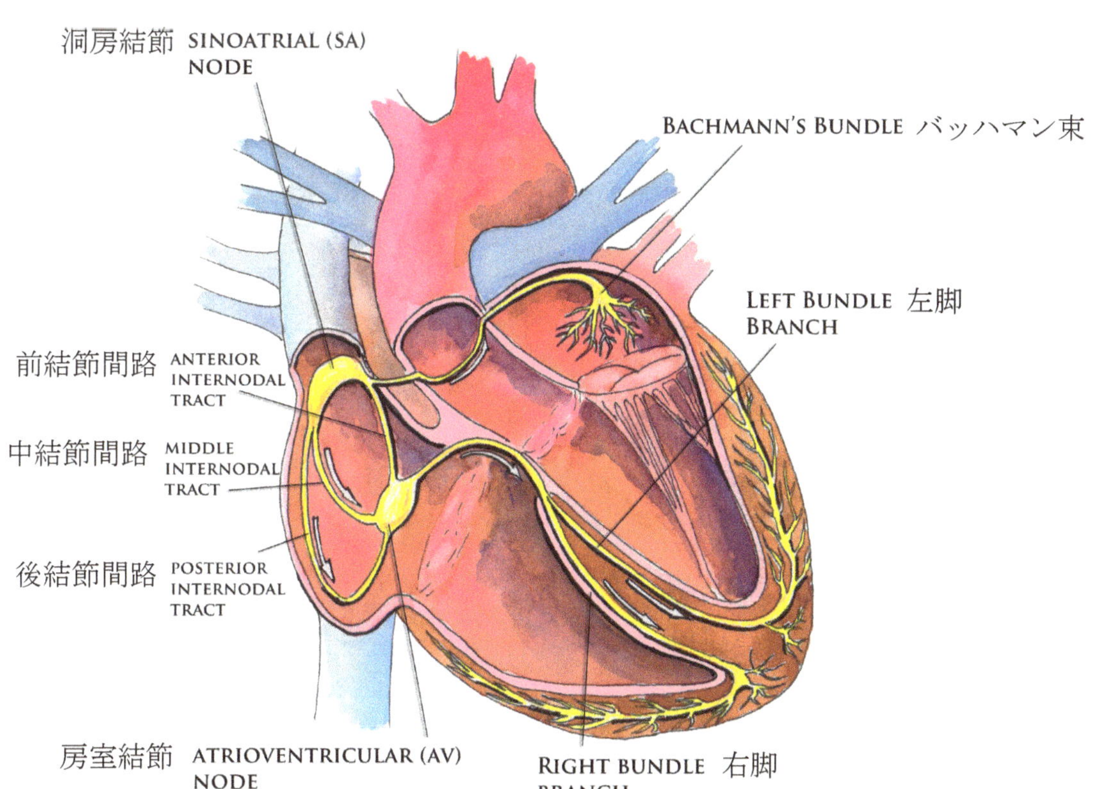

上大静脈 SUPERIOR VENA CAVA
AORTA 上大動脈
PULMONARY ARTERY 肺動脈
PULMONARY VEINS 肺静脈
LEFT ATRIUM 左心房
RIGHT ATRIUM 右心房
LEFT VENTRICLE 左心室
TRICUSPID VALVE 三尖弁
RIGHT VENTRICLE 右心室
INFERIOR VENA CAVA 下大静脈
洞房結節 SINOATRIAL (SA) NODE
BACHMANN'S BUNDLE バッハマン束
前結節間路 ANTERIOR INTERNODAL TRACT
LEFT BUNDLE 左脚 BRANCH
中結節間路 MIDDLE INTERNODAL TRACT
後結節間路 POSTERIOR INTERNODAL TRACT
房室結節 ATRIOVENTRICULAR (AV) NODE
RIGHT BUNDLE 右脚 BRANCH

CPR AND HEART FACTS
CPRと心臓の実態

DATA from AHA - Heart Disease and Stroke Statistics Update 2019
米国心臓協会（AHA）より － 心臓病と脳卒中の統計（2019年更新）

Cardiovascular Disease (CVD):
循環器疾患（CVD）：

Includes: coronary artery disease (CAD)
hypertension (HTN)
冠動脈疾患（CAD）、高血圧（HTN）を含む。

Congestive heart failure (CHF)
うっ血性心不全（CHF）
Strokes（CVA）脳卒中（CVA）

- CVD is the #1 cause of death, 1 in 3 deaths, or 840,000 per year.
  アメリカで1番多い死因は循環器疾患による － 年間84万人。

- 121.5 million Americans have some form of CVD.
  米国人の1億2150万人が、何らかの循環器疾患を抱えている。

- Men have higher incidence of CVD until age 65, then women have higher incidence.
  65歳までは男性の方が循環器疾患の発生率が高く、その後は女性の発生率の方が高い。

- 43.2% of all deaths in US in 2000 were due to CVD.
  米国において、2000年にあった死亡の原因の43.2%はCVDによるもの。

- Since 1900, CVD has been the #1 killer in US except for 1918.
  1900年以来、アメリカではCVDが死因の１位となっている（1918年を除く）。

- CVD claims more lives than next 5 leading causes of death combined.
  2〜6位までの死因よりも、CVDによる死者が多い。

CARDIOVASCULAR DISEASE TERMS:
循環器疾患(CVD)に関する用語

Arteriosclerosis: A disease of the arteries with thickening, hardening, and loss of elasticity in the arterial walls.
動脈硬化：動脈の内壁が厚くなったり、硬くなったりして本来の構造が壊れ、働きが悪くなる状態。

Atherosclerosis: The most common form of arteriosclerosis, marked by cholesterol-lipid-calcium deposits in arterial linings.
粥状動脈硬化(アテローム動脈硬化)：動脈硬化の中で最も多いパターン。動脈の内膜にコレステロールなどの脂肪からなるドロドロした粥状物質が溜まり、血管が部分的に狭くなる。

Coronary Artery Disease (CAD): Narrowing of coronary arteries sufficient to prevent adequate blood supply to the heart muscle.
冠動脈疾患(CAD)：冠状動脈が狭窄し、心筋への血液の供給が減少する病気。

Angina Pectoris: Pain around the heart caused by deficiency of blood supply to the heart.
狭心症：心臓に供給される血液が不足する為に胸部に痛みが起こる病気。

Myocardial Infarction: Condition caused by partial or complete occlusion of one of the coronary arteries.
心筋梗塞：冠動脈の急性閉塞による、心筋壊死が引き起こされる疾患。

Clinical Death: Patient without a pulse.
臨床死：心肺が停止した状態。

Biological Death: Occurs within 10 minutes of clinical death due to lack of oxygen to the brain.
脳死：脳への酸素の供給が行われなくなる為、臨床死後10分以内に起こる。

SUDDEN CARDIAC DEATH (SCD):
心臓突然死(SCD)：

When the heartbeat stops abruptly and un- expectedly, unassociated with any illness or injury.

病気や損傷に関係なく、突然心臓が止まって死に至る疾患。

Most common underlying cause of SCD is a heart attack that results in Ventricular Fibrillation (V-fib).

1番の原因とされているのは心室細動による心臓発作（V-fib）。

70 % of SCD occur at home, 18% in public settings, and 12% in nursing homes.

70%は自宅、18%は公共の場、12%は老人ホームにて発症。

Approximately 90% of SCD victims die before reaching hospital.

SCD患者の90%が病院に到着する前に死亡している。

Without bystander CPR success rates decline 7-10% every minute defibrillation is delayed.

現場でのCPRの成功率は、除細動器の到着が1分遅れる毎に、7-10%下がる。

Approximately 250,000 people die of coronary disease each year without ever being hospitalized.

毎年、約25万人の人が、病院に行く事なく心臓突然死により死亡している。

Causes of sudden death:
突然死の原因：

Sudden Cardiac Death – Cardiac Arrest Trauma
心臓突然死　－　主に心室細動による心停止。

Drowning
溺死

Asphyxiation
窒息

Electric Shock
感電

Allergic Reactions
アレルギー反応

RISK FACTORS FOR CARDIOVASCULAR DISEASE THAT CAN BE CHANGED:
変えることができる循環器疾患の危険因子：

CHOLESTEROL – LIPID PANEL:
コレステロール－脂質：

Total Cholesterol, HDL, LDL, and HDL/LDL ratios.

総コレステロール、HDLコレステロール、LDLコレステロール、HDL/LDLコレステロールの割合。

10% decrease in total cholesterol may result in 30% decrease in incidence of CVD.

総コレステロールが10%低下すると、循環器疾患の発症を30%抑えられると言われている。

Risk of heart attack greatest with Low High Density Lipoproteins (LDL) and high total cholesterol count (low HDL, high LDL).

LDLコレステロールと、高値の総コレステロールが、心臓発作のリスクを最大にする（HDLコレステロールが低く、LDLコレステロールが高いのがよくない状態）。

DIET AND OBESITY:
食生活と肥満

300,000 people die each year due to obesity related problems.

毎年、30万人が、肥満に起因する疾患で死亡している。

129 million people in American are overweight or obese, > 20% over ideal body weight.

1億2900万人のアメリカ人は、標準体重を20%以上超える太り過ぎ、肥満である。

61.2 million are obese (30.0Kg/m2).
6120万人は、肥満である（BMI 30.0kg/㎡）。

INACTIVITY:
運動不足

38.3% of Americans over-20-years old report ZERO leisure time physical activity.

20歳以上のアメリカ人の38.3%は、レジャーとしての運動を全く行っていないと報告されている。

SOLO ADULT CPR Skill Sheet:

What to Check for:	Skill to be demonstrated:
1. ASSESSES: Check for Responsiveness Check for Breathing	Shout "Are you OK?" If no response, apply painful stimuli. Check for no breathing or normal breathing.

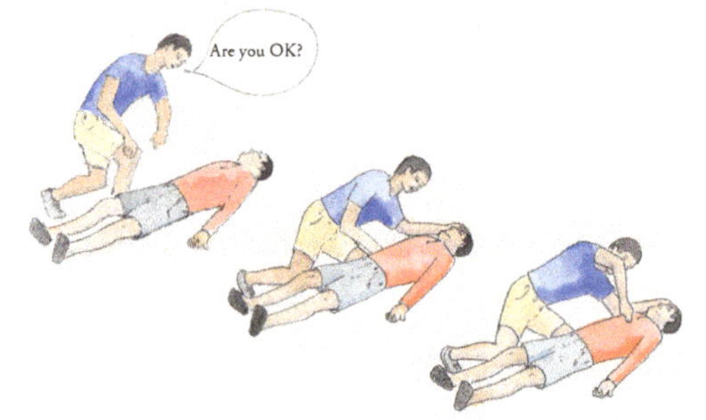

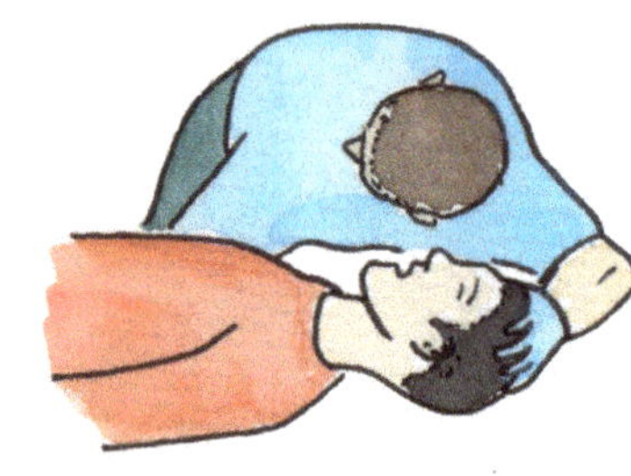

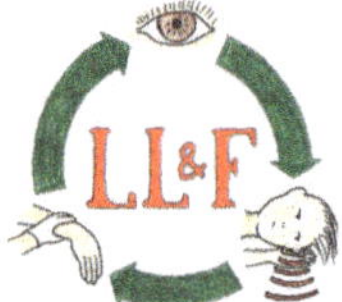

2. ACTIVATE:
Emergency Response System. Can use your cell phone to call for help.

Shout for help; direct someone to call for help.
Activate Emergency Response System and get an AED/defibrillator if available.

3. PULSE:
Check for pulse

Check for carotid pulse
(less than 10 seconds).

4. If there is a pulse but no breath sounds:
Start rescue breathing

Ventilate Patient once every 6 seconds, 10 breaths per minute.

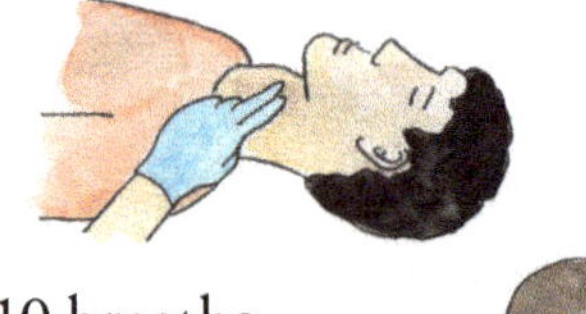

5. If there is no pulse: Start CPR.
Check for correct hand placement
Check for adequate rate.
Check for adequate depth
Allow for complete chest recoil
Minimize interruptions

Should begin compressions within 10 seconds of identifying cardiac arrest. Place one hand on the lower half of the sternum (with adults, place second hand on top of first).
Compress the chest at least 2 inches (5cm or 1/3 body depth), but not greater than 2.4 inches (6cm) 30 times in 20 seconds (1 1/2 times per second) allowing chest to fully recoil.
Follow with 2 rescue breaths. (Each breath delivered over one second, each causing the chest to rise).
Continue 30 compressions followed by 2 breaths (Use the same ratio for either one rescuer or two).

6. If no AED is available, continue CPR for 5 cycles of 30:2, stopping every five cycles to check for pulse.

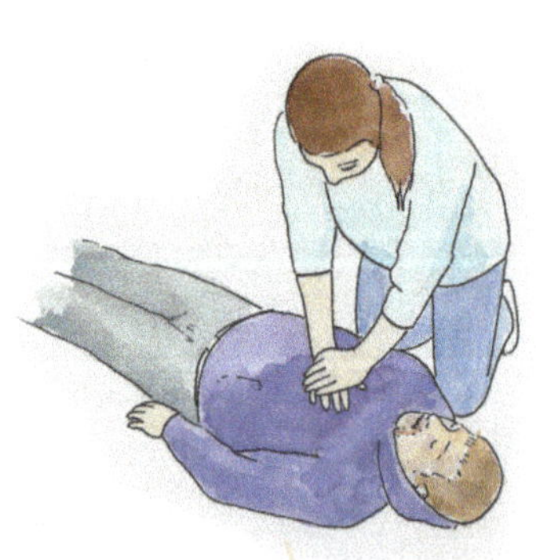

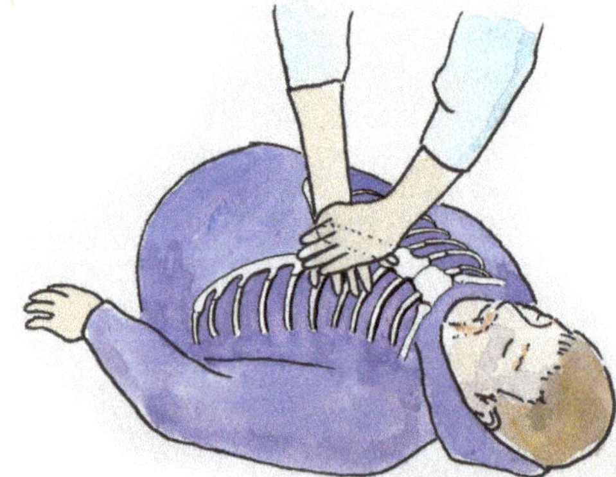

SOLO 成人CPRスキルシート

チェック項目	実施する技術
1. 評価 応答の確認 呼吸の確認	"大丈夫ですか？"と問いかける 反応が無い場合、痛みの刺激を与える。 呼吸の有無、もしくは普通に呼吸しているか。 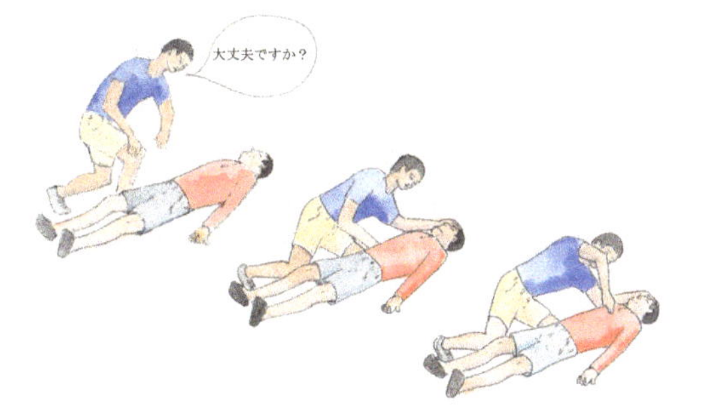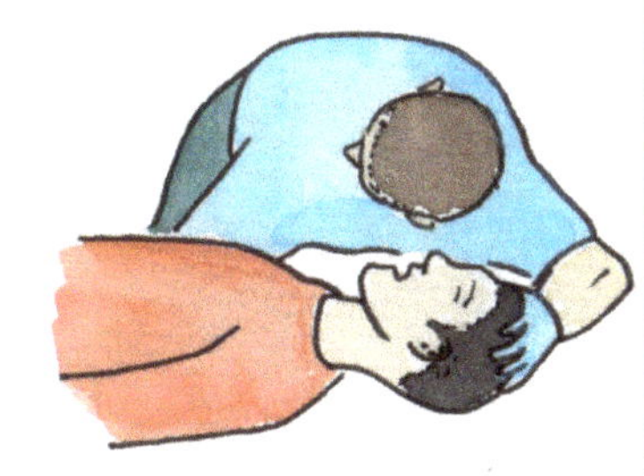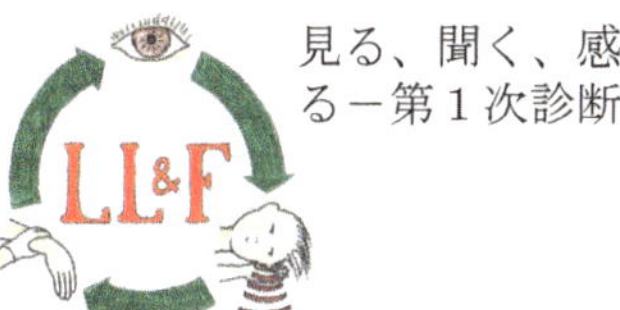
2. 始動 緊急対応システム。 携帯電話にて救助の要請。	助けを呼ぶ；助けを呼ぶよう指示をする。緊急対応システムの始動と可能であればAEDの手配をする。
3. 脈拍 脈拍の確認	頚動脈の脈拍の確認（10秒以上）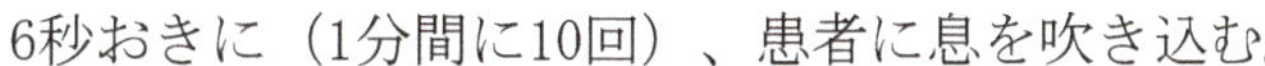
4. 脈拍はあるが、呼吸音がない場合：人工呼吸を始める	6秒おきに（1分間に10回）、患者に息を吹き込む。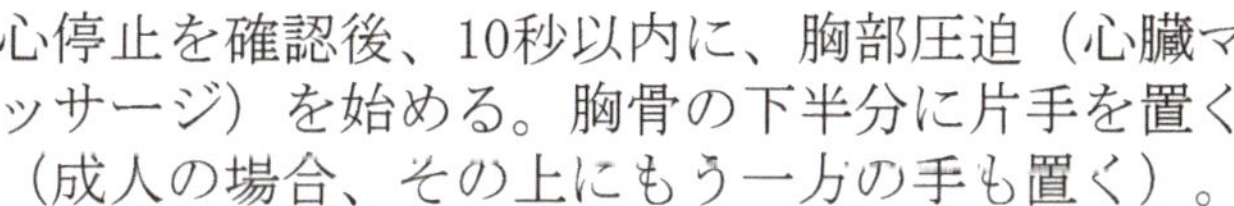
5. 脈拍がない場合：CPRを始める 手を置く位置の確認。 適切な速さの確認。 適切な深度の確認。 胸壁が元の高さに戻るのを確認する。 できる限り、中断しない。	心停止を確認後、10秒以内に、胸部圧迫（心臓マッサージ）を始める。胸骨の下半分に片手を置く（成人の場合、その上にもう一方の手も置く）。 少なくとも5cm（または胸の厚さの1/3）胸部を圧迫するが、6cmを超えないようにする。20秒に30回（毎秒1.5回）で、胸壁の高さが戻るように。 その後、人工呼吸を2回（1回1秒以上、胸部が挙上） 胸部圧迫30回、人工呼吸2回を繰り返す（救助者が1人でも2人でも、同様の回数）。
6.AEDがない場合 胸部圧迫30回、人工呼吸2回のCPRを5セット行う毎に、脈拍を確認する。	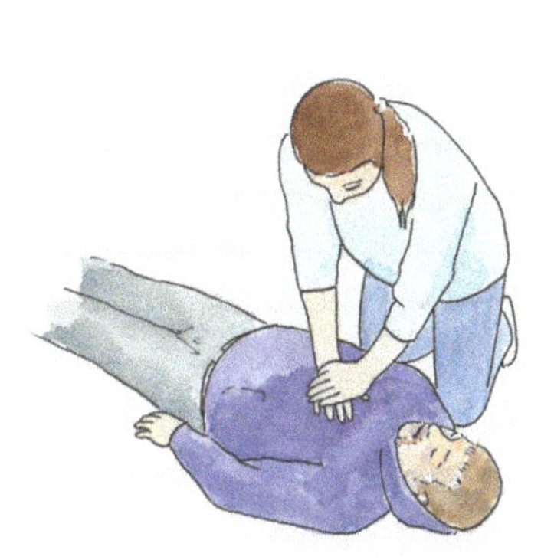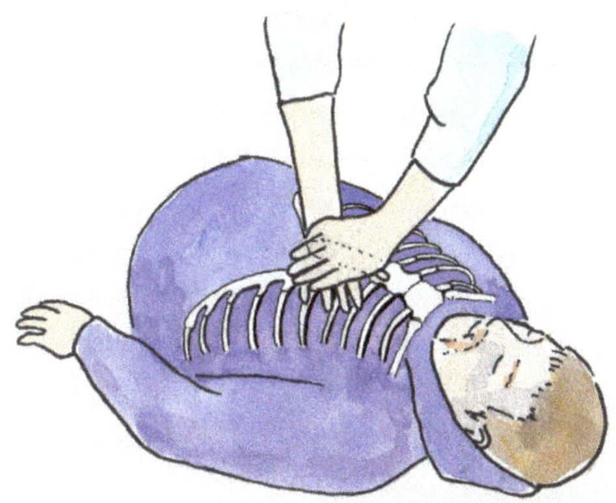

SOLO ADULT CPR Skill Sheet:

What to Check for:	Skill to be demonstrated:
7. **AED and CPR**	Apply and use AED as soon as it arrives.
8. **AED**	Turn on AED. Place proper size pads in correct locations. Clear patient and allow AED to analyze rhythm. If advised by AED, clear patient and deliver a shock. Resume CPR immediately after shock delivery. Do not turn off AED during CPR. ***If shock not advised***, check for pulse. If no pulse, resume CPR, five cycles of 30:2

9. **After 5 cycles (approximately 2 minutes) of 30 compressions to 2 breaths, stop CPR and let AED re-analyze.**	After approximately 2 minutes the AED will tell you to stop CPR so it can analyze the rhythm. Follow prompts from the AED.
	   If 'Shock advised," repeat step **8**, re-shock and continue CPR.
	   If "no shock advised," reassess patient for pulse and breathing.

10. **If no pulse: Start 5 additional cycles of 30 compressions and 2 breaths.**	See step **8**.
11. **If pulse: Reassess for adequate breathing**	Reassess for adequate breathing; continue rescue breathing if necessary.
12. **If there is a pulse, but inadequate breathing:**	Continue rescue breathing.
13. **If there is a pulse and adequate breathing:**	Monitor until help arrives.

チェック項目	実施する技術
7. AEDとCPR	AED到着後、ただちに装着し使用する。
8. AED	AEDの電源を入れる。 適切なサイズのパッドを、正しい位置に貼る。 患者から離れ、AEDに心電図を解析させる。 AEDの指示があれば、患者から離れ、電気ショックを与える。その後、直ちにCPRを再開する。 CPR中、AEDの電源は切らない。 **電気ショックの指示がない場合は、**脈拍を確認する。脈拍がない場合は、CPRを再開する（胸部圧迫30回、人工呼吸2回を5セット）。
9. 胸部圧迫30回、人工呼吸2回を5セット（約2分間）行った後、CPRを中断して、再び、AEDに解析させる。	約2分後、AEDよりCPRを中止するよう指示があり、AEDが心電図を解析する。AEDの指示に従う。 電気ショックの指示がある場合、8を繰り返す。再度ショックを与え、CPRを続ける。 電気ショックの指示がない場合、再度、患者の脈拍と呼吸を再評価する。
10.脈拍がない場合：胸部圧迫30回、人工呼吸2回を5セット追加する。	**手順8を参照。**
11. 脈拍がある場合：適切な呼吸の再評価	適切な呼吸かどうか再評価する；必要があれば、人工呼吸を継続する。
12. 脈拍はあるが、呼吸が十分でない場合：	人工呼吸を継続する。
13. 脈拍と十分な呼吸がある場合：	救助が到着するまで、観察を続ける。

SOLO CHILD CPR Skill Sheet:
(1-Year-old to puberty)

What to Check for:	Skill to be demonstrated:
1. ASSESSES: Check for Responsiveness. Check for Breathing. **If you witnessed collapse:** Follow steps for adult. **If you did not witness collapse:** Give 2 minutes CPR, then get help and AED.	Shout "Are you OK?" If no response, apply painful stimuli. Check for no breathing or normal breathing. 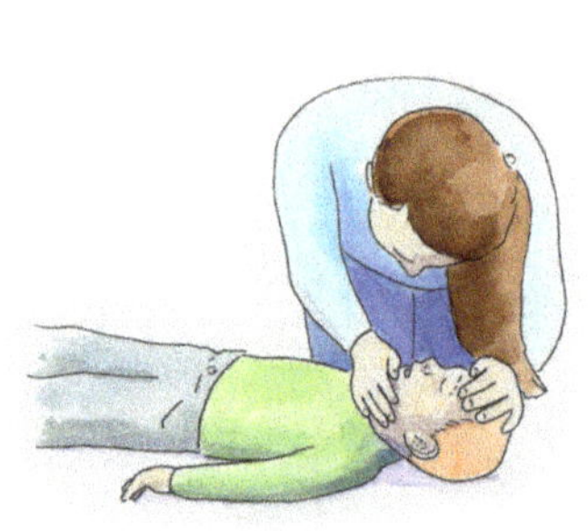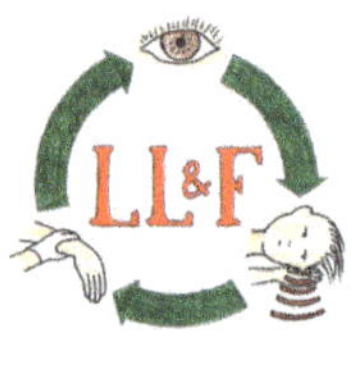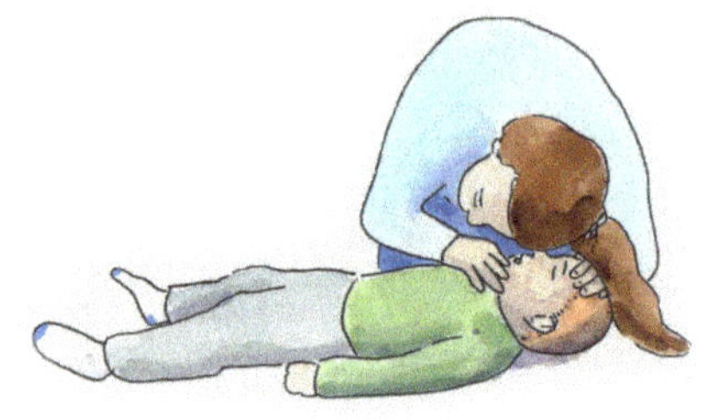
2. ACTIVATE: Emergency response system if you have two rescuers or a second person on scene. If you are the only rescuer activate after 2 minutes CPR.	Shout for help; direct someone to call for help. Activate Emergency Response System and get an AED/defibrillator if available.
3. PULSE: Check for pulse.	Check for cartotid pulse (less than 10 seconds). 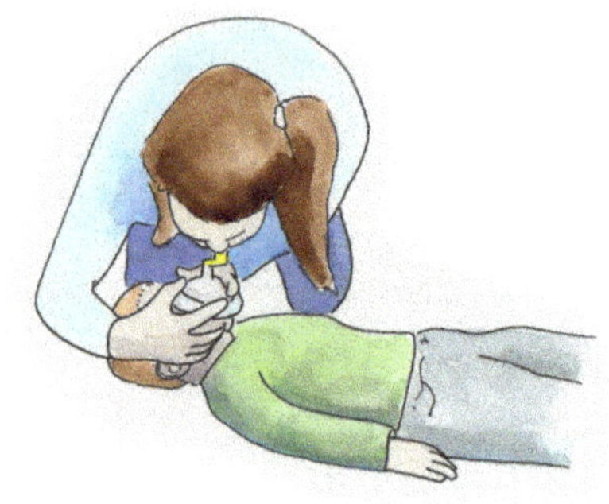
4. If there is a pulse but no breath sounds: Start rescue breathing.	Ventilate Patient once every 3-5 seconds, 12 breaths per minute.
5. If there is no pulse: Start CPR. Check for Correct hand placement. Check for adequate rate. Check for adequate depth. Allow for complete chest recoil. Minimize interruptions. Activate ERS if you have not already done so.	Begin compressions within 10 seconds of identifying cardiac arrest. Place one or two hands on lower half of patient's sternum. Compress the chest at least 2 inches (5cm, or 1/3 body depth) 30 times in 20 seconds, allowing chest to fully recoil. Follow with 2 rescue breaths. One rescuer: Continue 30 compressions followed by 2 breaths. Two rescuers: Continue 15 compressions followed by 2 breaths.

SOLO 小児CPRスキルシート：
（1歳〜思春期）

チェック項目	実施する技術
1. 評価 応答の確認 呼吸の確認	"大丈夫ですか？"と問いかける 反応が無い場合、痛みの刺激を与える。 呼吸の有無、もしくは普通に呼吸しているか。 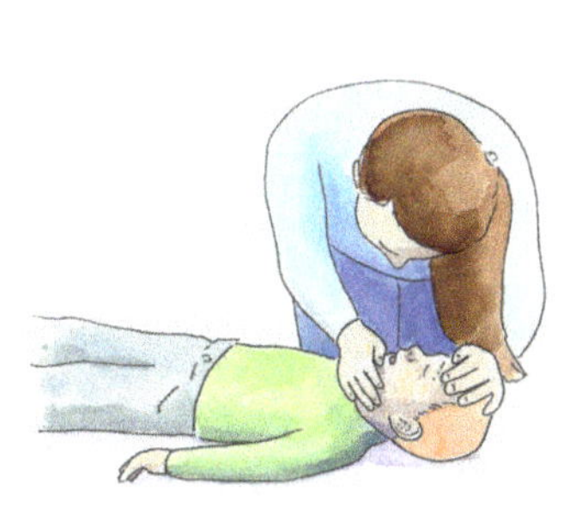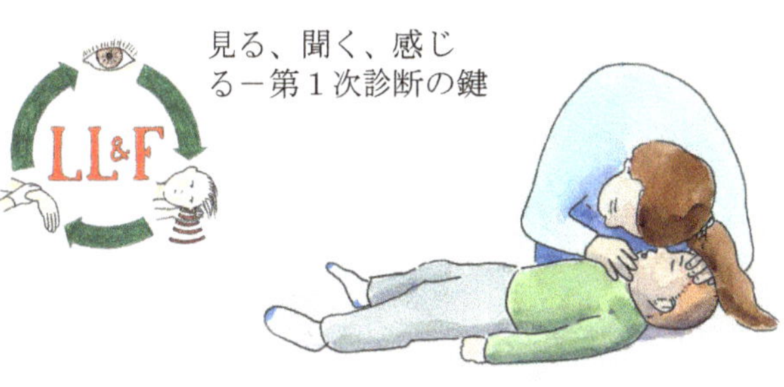
倒れる場面を目撃した場合: 成人の手順を参照。 **倒れる場面を見ていない場合:** AED. 2分間CPRを実施し、その後、助けを呼び、AEDを手配。	
2. 始動 緊急対応システム。 携帯電話にて救助の要請。 救助者が2名またはその場にもう1人いる場合、緊急対応システムに通報する。他に救助者がいない場合は、2分間のCPRの後に通報する。	助けを呼ぶ；助けを呼ぶよう指示をする。緊急対応システムの始動と可能であればAEDの手配をする。
3. 脈拍 脈拍の確認	頚動脈の脈拍の確認（10秒以上） 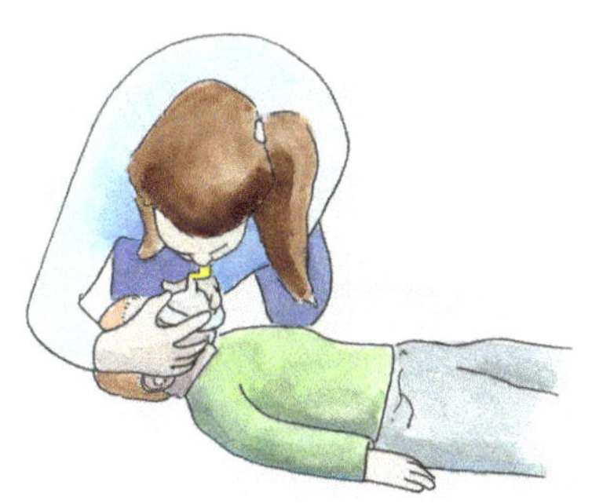
4. 脈拍はあるが、呼吸音がない場合: 人工呼吸を始める	3-5秒おきに（1分間に12回）、患者に息を吹き込む。
5. 脈拍がない場合:CPRを始める 手を置く位置の確認。 適切な速さの確認。 適切な深度の確認。 胸壁が元の高さに戻るのを確認する。 できる限り、中断しない。 まだ連絡していなければ、緊急対応システムに通報する。	心停止を確認後、10秒以内に、胸部圧迫（心臓マッサージ）を始める。 胸骨の下半分に片手または両手を置く。 少なくとも5cm（または胸の厚さの1/3）胸部を圧迫する。20秒に30回で、胸壁の高さが戻るように。 その後、人工呼吸を2回。 救助者1名の場合：胸部圧迫30回、人工呼吸2回を繰り返す。 救助者2名の場合：胸部圧迫15回、人工呼吸2回を繰り返す。

SOLO CHILD CPR Skill Sheet:
(1-Year-old to puberty)

What to Check for:	Skill to be demonstrated:
6. AED and CPR	Apply and use AED as soon as it arrives.
7. AED	Turn on AED. Place proper size pads in correct locations. Clear patient and allow AED to analyze rhythm. If advised by AED, clear patient and deliver a shock. Resume CPR immediately after shock delivery. Do not turn off AED during CPR. ***If shock not advised***, check for pulse. If no pulse resume CPR five cycles of 30:2
8. After 5 cycles (approximately 2 minutes) of 30 compressions to 2 breaths, reassess for pulse	After approximately 2 minutes the AED will tell you to stop CPR so it can analyze the rhythm. Follow prompts from the AED. If 'Shock advised," repeat step **7,** re-shock and continue CPR. If "no shock advised," reassess patient for pulse and breathing.
9. If no pulse: **Start 5 additional cycles of 30 compressions and 2 breaths**	See step **7.**
10. If pulse: Reassess for adequate breathing	Reassess for adequate breathing; continue rescue breathing If necessary.
11. If there is a pulse, but inadequate breathing:	Continue rescue breathing once every 3-5 seconds.
12. If there is a pulse and adequate breathing:	Monitor until help arrives.

チェック項目	実施する技術
6. AED and CPR	AED到着後、ただちに装着し使用する。
7.AED	AEDの電源を入れる。 適切なサイズのパッドを、正しい位置に貼る。 患者から離れ、AEDに心電図を解析させる。 AEDの指示があれば、患者から離れ、電気ショックを与える。その後、直ちにCPRを再開する。 CPR中、AEDの電源は切らない。 **電気ショックの指示がない場合は、**脈拍を確認する。脈拍がない場合は、CPRを再開する（胸部圧迫30回、人工呼吸2回を5セット）。
8. 胸部圧迫30回、人工呼吸2回を5セット（約2分間）行った後、脈拍を再評価する。	約2分後、AEDよりCPRを中止するよう指示があり、AEDが心電図を解析する。AEDの指示に従う。 電気ショックの指示がある場合、7を繰り返す。再度ショックを与え、CPRを続ける。 電気ショックの指示がない場合、再度、患者の脈拍と呼吸を再評価する。
9. 脈拍がない場合：胸部圧迫30回、人工呼吸2回を5セット追加する。	手順7を参照。
10. 脈拍がある場合：十分な呼吸の再評価	十分な呼吸かどうか再評価する；必要があれば、人工呼吸を継続する。
11. 脈拍はあるが、呼吸が十分でない場合：	3-5秒おきに人工呼吸を継続する。
12. 脈拍と十分な呼吸がある場合：	救助が到着するまで、観察を続ける。

SOLO INFANT CPR Skill Sheet:
(0-12 months-old)

What to Check for:	Skill to be demonstrated:
1. ASSESSES: Check for Responsiveness Check for Breathing.	Tickle bottom of infant's foot to check for responsiveness. If unresponsive, check to see if infant is breathing.
2. ACTIVATE: Emergency response system if you have two rescuers or a second person on scene. If you are the only rescuer activate after 2 minutes CPR.	Shout for help; direct someone to call for help. Activate Emergency Response System.
3. PULSE: Check for pulse.	Check for a brachial pulse (not carotid). 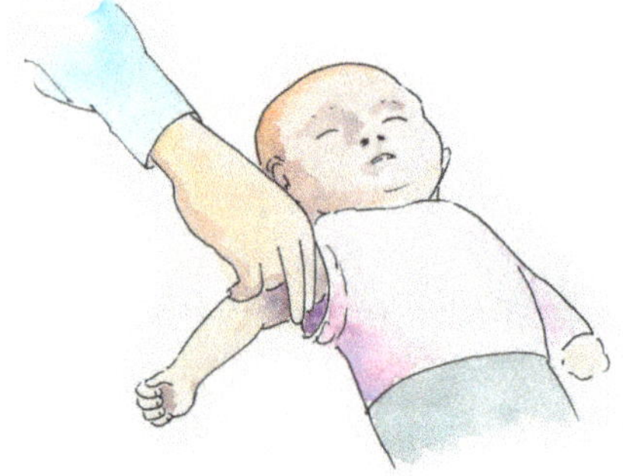
4. If there is a pulse but no breath sounds: Start rescue breathing.	Ventilate Patient once every 3-5 seconds, 12-20 breaths per minute.
5. If there is no pulse: Start CPR. Check for Correct hand placement. Check for adequate rate. Check for adequate depth. Allow for complete chest recoil. Minimize interruptions. **Compression to ventilation ratios: One Rescuer CPR** Activate EMS if you have not already done so.	Begin compressions within 10 seconds of identifying cardiac arrest. Place two fingers just below the nipple line. Compress the chest 1/3 depth of the chest (aprox 1 ½ inches, or 4cm) 30 times in 20 seconds, allowing chest to fully recoil. Follow with 2 rescue breaths. 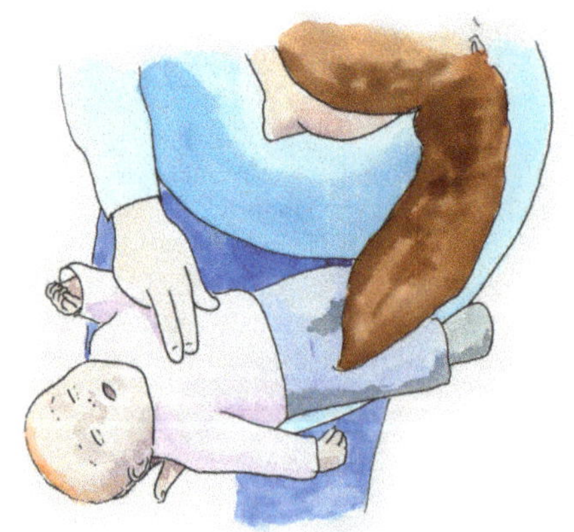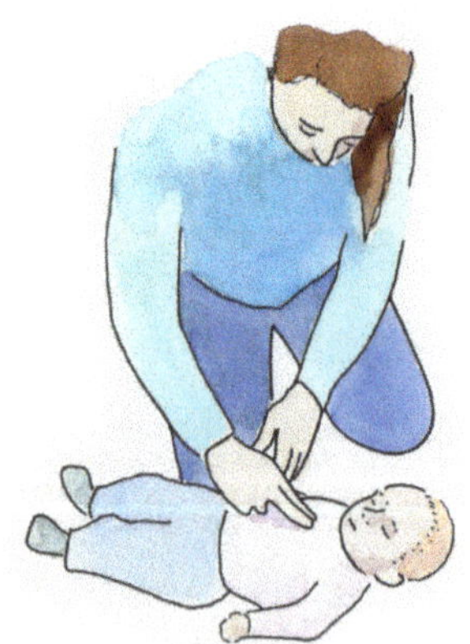 One Rescuer CPR: 30 compressions to 2 breaths, 2 fingers at the nipple line.

SOLO 乳児CPRスキルシート：
（新生児〜1歳未満）

チェック項目	実施する技術
1.評価 応答の確認 呼吸の確認	乳児の足底をくすぐり、反応を確認する。 反応がなければ、呼吸を確認する。
2.始動 救助者が2名またはその場にもう一人いる場合、緊急対応システムに通報する。他に救助者がいない場合は、2分間のCPRの後に通報する。	助けを呼ぶ；助けを呼ぶよう指示をする。緊急対応システムの始動と可能であればAEDの手配をする。
3. 脈拍 脈拍の確認	上腕の脈拍を確認する （頚動脈ではなく）。
4. 脈拍はあるが、呼吸音がない場合： 人工呼吸を始める	3-5秒おきに（1分間に12-20回）、患者に息を吹き込む。
5. 脈拍がない場合：CPRを始める 手を置く位置の確認。 適切な速さの確認。 適切な深度の確認。 胸壁が元の高さに戻るのを確認する。 できる限り、中断しない。	心停止を確認後、10秒以内に、胸部圧迫（心臓マッサージ）を始める。 乳頭を結ぶラインのすぐ下に、2本の指を置く。 胸の厚さの1/3（約4cm）、胸部を圧迫する。20秒に30回で、胸壁の高さが戻るように。 その後、人工呼吸を2回。
圧迫と人工呼吸の比：救助者1名のCPR まだ連絡していなければ、緊急対応システムに通報する。	救助者1名のCPR：胸部圧迫30回、人工呼吸2回。乳頭を結ぶラインを2本指で。

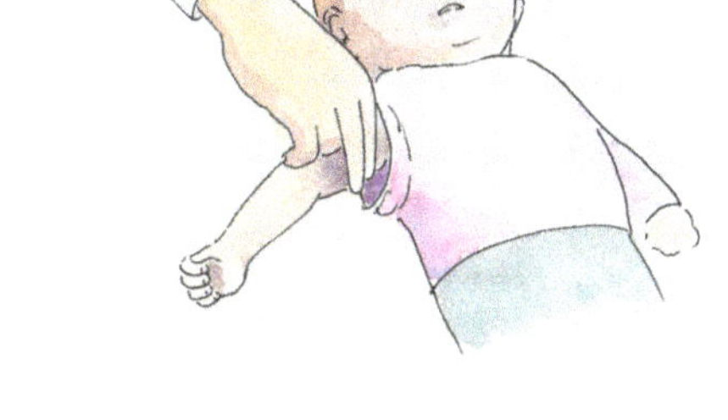

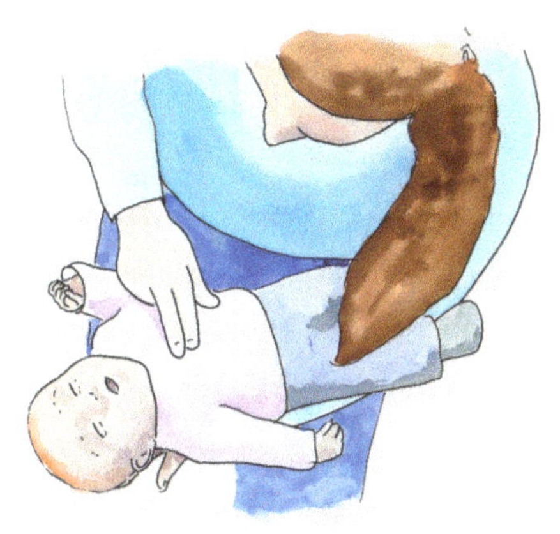

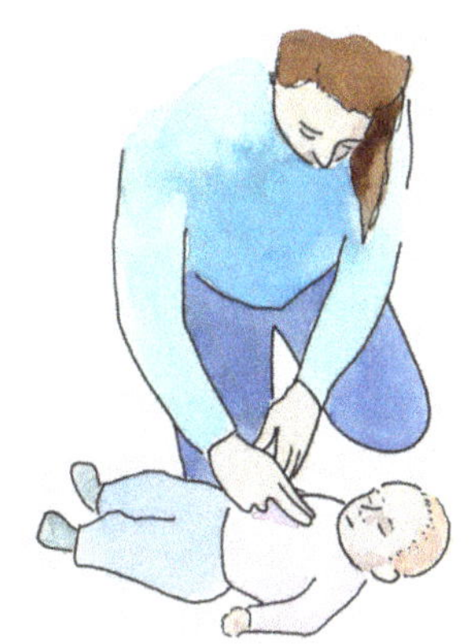

What to Check for:	Skill to be demonstrated:
Compression to ventilation ratios: Two Rescuer CPR	Two Rescuer CPR: 15 compressions to 2 breaths, thumb encircling chest method at nipple line.
6. After 5 cycles (approximately 2 minutes) of 30 compressions to 2 breaths, or 15 compressions to 2 breaths, reassess for pulse.	Check for brachial pulse for at least 5 seconds, but not more than 10 seconds.
7. If no pulse, begin five additional cycles of 30:2 or 15:2 ratio of compressions to breaths.	See step **6**.
8. If pulse: Reassess for adequate breathing.	Look for chest rise, listen and feel for air movement.
9. If there is a pulse, but inadequate breathing:	Continue rescue breathing; ventilate once every 3-5 seconds.
10. If there is a pulse and adequate breathing:	Monitor until help arrives.

SOLO 乳児CPRスキルシート：
（新生児〜1歳未満）

チェック項目	実施する技術
圧迫と人工呼吸の比：救助者2名のCPR	救助者2名のCPR：胸部圧迫15回、人工呼吸2回。胸部の乳頭を結ぶラインを親指で囲む手法で。
6. 胸部圧迫30回、人工呼吸2回を5セット、または、胸部圧迫15回、人工呼吸2回を5セット（約2分間）行った後、脈拍を再評価する。	少なくとも5秒間（但し10秒を超えない）、上腕の脈拍を確認する。
7. 脈拍がない場合、胸部圧迫30回＆人工呼吸2回、または、胸部圧迫15回＆人工呼吸2回を5セット追加する。	手順6を参照。
8. 脈拍がある場合：適切な呼吸の再評価	胸部の挙上を目視、呼吸音を聞き、空気の動きを感じる。
9. 脈拍はあるが、呼吸が十分でない場合：	人工呼吸を継続する；3-5秒に1回息を吹き込む。
10. 脈拍と十分な呼吸がある場合：	救助が到着するまで、観察を続ける。

SOLO FOREIGN-BODY AIRWAY OBSTRUCTION
ADULT AND CHILD SKILL SHEET
(1 year of age and older)

What to Check for:	Skill to be demonstrated:
1. Assess for airway obstruction	Poor or no air exchange, increased respiratory difficulty, possible cyanosis of the lips and nail beds (bluish), universal choking sign.
2. Position patient for abdominal thrusts	Stand behind the patient and wrap your arms around the patient's waist. Place the thumb side of your fist against the patient's abdomen, midline, above the navel and well below the sternum.
	Position for adult *Position for child*
3. Deliver abdominal thrusts	Grasp your fist with your other hand and force both hands together into the patient's abdomen with a quick, forceful upward thrust.

SOLO 気道異物除去スキルシート：
（1歳以上）

チェック項目	実施する技術
1. 気道の異物を評価	換気が非常に乏しいか、全くなく、呼吸困難が増強。唇と爪のチアノーゼ（青紫になる）。世界共通のチョークサイン。
2. 患者を腹部突き上げ法の姿勢にする。	患者の後ろに立ち、ウエスト付近に手を回す。 握りこぶしを作り、親指側を、患者の腹部中央、へその上方で、みぞおちよりも十分下方に当てる。
3. 腹部を突き上げる	もう片方の手で、握りこぶしをしっかり握り、両手で素早く患者の腹部を手前上方に押す。

SOLO FOREIGN-BODY AIRWAY OBSTRUCTION
ADULT AND CHILD SKILL SHEET
(1 year of age and older)

What to Check for:	Skill to be demonstrated:
4. **Repeat thrusts**	Repeat thrusts until object is expelled from the airway or until patient becomes unconscious. Give each thrust as a separate and distinct movement to dislodge the obstruction.
5. **Obese or pregnant**	Perform chest thrusts instead of abdominal thrusts.

If the patient becomes unresponsive:

What to Check for:	Skill to be demonstrated:
1. **Activate the Emergency Response system:**	Send someone to call for help, but do not leave the patient alone.
2. **Begin CPR:** **30 compressions to 2 rescue breaths.**	Lower the patient to the ground and begin chest compressions. Each time you go to give ventilations, open the patient's mouth and look inside for the obstructing object. If the object is visible, remove if possible.
3. **After 5 cycles of 30 compressions and 2 rescue breaths, check that the Emergency Response System has been activated.**	Check that Emergency Medical help has been notified and continue CPR. Remember to look in the airway before giving rescue breaths.

SOLO 乳児CPRスキルシート：
（新生児〜1歳未満）

チェック項目	実施する技術
4. 腹部突き上げを繰り返す。	気道から異物が取れるか、患者の意識がなくなるまで、腹部突き上げ法を継続する。 突き上げは、異物を取り除くために、1回ずつのはっきりした動きとして行う。
5. 肥満または妊婦	腹部突き上げ法の代わりに、胸部突き上げ法を実施する。

患者の反応がなくなった場合：

チェック項目	実施する技術
1. 緊急対応システムに通報する。	誰かに助けを呼びに行かせる。ただし、患者を1人にしない。
2. CPRを開始する： 胸部圧迫30回、人工呼吸2回	患者を地面に寝かせ、胸部圧迫を始める。 人工呼吸のたびに、患者の口を開けて、異物が口を塞いでいないか目視する。 異物が見える場合、可能であれば取り除く。
3. 胸部圧迫30回、人工呼吸2回を5セット行った後、緊急対応システムと連絡が取れているか確認する。	緊急対応システムと連絡が取れたかを確認し、CPRを継続する。人工呼吸をする前に、忘れずに気道を目視する。

SOLO FOREIGN-BODY AIRWAY OBSTRUCTION
INFANT SKILL SHEET
(0-12 months old)

What to Check for:	Skill to be demonstrated:
1. Assess for airway obstruction.	Poor or no air exchange, increased respiratory difficulty, possible cyanosis of the lips and nail beds (bluish), inability to cry.
2. Position patient for back slaps.	Kneel or sit with the infant in your lap. Hold the infant facedown resting on your forearm with the head slightly lower than the chest. Support the infant's head and jaw with your hand. Rest your arm on your leg or lap to support the infant.
3. Deliver 5 back slaps.	Slap the infant forcefully in the middle of the back between the shoulder blades using the heel of your hand.
4. Position the infant for chest thrusts	Place your free hand on the infant's back supporting the back of the head with the palm of your hand. The infant should be cradled between your two forearms. Turn the infant as a unit while carefully supporting the head and neck. Hold the infant on its back with your forearm resting on your lap or thigh. 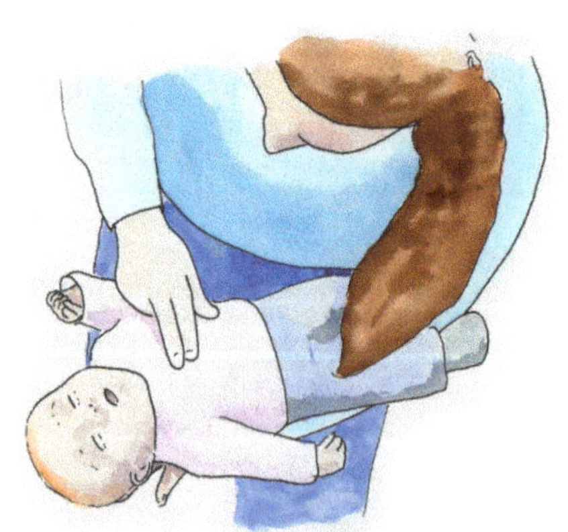

SOLO 気道異物除去スキルシート：
（新生児〜1歳未満）

チェック項目	実施する技術
1. 気道の異物を評価	換気が非常に乏しいか、全くなく、呼吸困難が増強。唇と爪のチアノーゼ（青紫になる）。泣くことができない。
2. 乳児を背部叩打法の姿勢にする。	乳児を膝に乗せ、膝を曲げるか座る。 乳児をうつ伏せにして、頭が胸部より低くなるように、上腕に乗せる。 乳児の頭と顎を手で支える。 乳児を支えるため、腕を太腿か膝に置く。
3. 背中を5回叩打する。	乳児の背部（肩甲骨の間）を、手のひらの基部で強く叩く。
4. 乳児を胸部圧迫が出来る態勢にする。	空いている手を乳児の背中に置き、手のひらで乳児の後頭部を支える。 乳児は、両腕の上腕で抱えられている状態である。 乳児の頭部と頸部をしっかり支えながら、仰向けにする。 上腕を太腿か膝に置き、乳児を仰向けに抱える。

SOLO FOREIGN-BODY AIRWAY OBSTRUCTION
INFANT SKILL SHEET
(0-12 months old)

What to Check for:	Skill to be demonstrated:
5. Deliver up to 5 chest thrusts.	Provide up to 5 quick downward chest thrusts in the same place as chest compressions. Deliver chest thrusts at a rate of 1 per second.
6. Repeat until the object is removed or the infant becomes unresponsive.	Continue the sequence of 5 back slaps and up to 5 chest thrusts.

If the patient becomes unresponsive:

What to Check for:	Skill to be demonstrated:
1. Activate the Emergency Response system.	Send someone to call for help, but do not leave the patient alone.
2. Begin CPR with one extra step.	Each time you open the airway, look for the obstructing object in the back of the throat. If the object is visible, remove if possible.
3. After 5 cycles, check that the Emergency Response System has been activated.	Check that Emergency Medical help has been notified and continue CPR. Remember to look in the airway before giving rescue breaths.

SOLO 気道異物除去スキルシート：
（新生児〜1歳未満）

チェック項目	実施する技術
5. 胸部を押す（最大で5回まで）。	胸部圧迫（心配蘇生）と同じ場所を素早く押す（最大で5回、1秒に1回の早さで）。
6. 異物が取れるか、乳児の反応がなくなるまで繰り返す。	背部叩打法5回と胸部圧迫を最大5回を繰り返す。

患者の反応がなくなった場合：

チェック項目	実施する技術
1. 緊急対応システムに通報する。	誰かに助けを呼びに行かせる。ただし、患者を1人にしない。
2. 手順を追加したCPRを開始する。	気道を確保するたびに、患者の口を開けて、異物が喉の奥を塞いでいないか目視する。異物が見える場合、可能であれば取り除く。
3. 5セット行った後、緊急対応システムと連絡が取れているか確認する。	緊急対応システムと連絡が取れたかを確認し、CPRを継続する。人工呼吸をする前に、忘れずに気道を目視する。

SUMMARY OF BASIC LIFE SUPPORT

Action	Adult:	Child:	Infant:
AIRWAY	Head tilt chin lift		Neutral in-line position
BREATHING	2 breaths at 1 breath per second	2 effective breaths at 1 breath per second.	
Rescue breathing without compressions	1 breath every 5 seconds: 10-12 breaths per minute	1 every 3-5 seconds: 15-20 breaths per minute	
Rescue breaths for CPR with advanced airway	Adults 30 compressions to 2 breaths, approximately 10 breaths per minute	Children and infants, One Rescuer CPR: same rate as adult. Children and infants, Two rescuer CPR: 15 Compressions to 2 breaths.	
Foreign-body Airway obstruction (Conscious patient)	Abdominal thrusts Chest thrusts if obese or pregnant		Back slaps and chest thrusts
Foreign-body Airway obstruction (Unconscious patient)	If patient becomes unconscious from choking, activate the Emergency Response System and begin CPR. Each time you open the airway to ventilate, check throat and mouth for foreign objects.		
CIRCULATION Pulse check 10 seconds	Carotid		Brachial
Compression landmarks	Lower half of sternum		Just below nipple line
Compression method	With fist covered by other hand, thrust hard and fast. Allow complete recoil.		1 rescuer CPR: 2 or 3 fingers 2 rescuer CPR: 2 thumbs encircling chest technique
Compression depth	At least 2 inches	2 inches	1 ½ inches
Compression rate	Approximately 100/120 compressions per minute		
Compression to ventilation ratio	30:2 one or two rescuer	Children and infants—one rescuer 30:2 Children and infants—two rescuer 15:2	
Two-rescuer CPR	One rescuer ventilates; one rescuer does compressions. Switch every two minutes. Switch should take less than 5 seconds.		Same as for child or adult using thumbs–encircling-chest method
DEFIBRILLATION AED	Use adult pads. Do not use child pads.	Use AED after 5 cycles of CPR. Use pediatric system if available.	No recommendations for infant less than one year of age

救命の基本サマリー

行動	成人	子ども	乳児
気道確保	頭部後屈、下顎挙上		平らに寝かせる
呼吸の確認	2回息を吹き込む（1回/秒）	2回効果的に息を吹き込む（1回/秒）	
人工呼吸（胸部圧迫なし）	5秒に1回（10-12回/分）	3-5秒に1回（15-20回/分）	
人工呼吸（CPRと高度な気道確保）	胸部圧迫30回に、人工呼吸2回（約10呼吸/分）	救助者1名：胸部圧迫30回に人工呼吸2回 救助者2名：胸部圧迫15回に人工呼吸2回	
気道異物除去（意識のある患者）	腹部突き上げ法 肥満または妊婦：胸部圧迫		背部叩打法と 胸部圧迫
気道異物除去（意識のない患者）	患者が窒息により意識を失った場合は、緊急対応システムを始動し、CPRを開始する。 人工呼吸の為、気道を確保するたびに、口と喉に異物がないか確認する。		
循環の確認 脈拍を10秒間確認	頸部		上腕
圧迫をする所	胸骨の下半分		乳頭を結ぶラインの真下
圧迫方法	重ねた両手で、強く早く圧迫する。胸壁の高さを元に戻す。		救助者1名のCPR：2本指で。 救助者2名のCPR：胸部を親指で囲む手法で。
圧迫の深さ	少なくとも5cm	5cm	4cm
圧迫の早さ	約100-120回/分		
圧迫と人工呼吸の比	胸部圧迫30回：人工呼吸2回 救助者1名でも2名でも	子どもと乳児 救助者1名　胸部圧迫30回：人工呼吸2回 救助者2名　胸部圧迫15回：人工呼吸2回	
救助者2名のCPR	人工呼吸と胸部圧迫を各1名で行う。2分毎に交代する（交代は5秒以内で素早く）		成人＆子どもと同様。胸部を親指で囲む手法
除細動　AED	成人用パッドを使用（小児用は使用しない）	CPR5セットの後、AEDを使用する（あれば小児用システムを使用）	1歳未満の乳児には、使用しない。

CPR CONSIDERATIONS IN THE REMOTE ENVIRONMENT
ウィルダネスでのCPRの考察

When to begin CPR:
いつCPRを開始するか:

Street and Wilderness: For any pulseless individuals.
道路＆ウィルダネス：脈拍がない人がいる場合

EXCEPTION: Do NOT begin CPR if:
例外：CPRを開始しないケース:

Street:
道路:

Scene is unsafe.
現場が安全ではない場合

Rigor mortis is present.
死後硬直がある場合

Dependent lividity is present.
死斑が認められる場合

Injuries are incompatible with life.
生存不可能な損傷

DNR orders are present.
蘇生処置拒否の指示がある場合

Putrefaction (rot) is evident.
腐敗が明らかな場合

Wilderness:
ウィルダネス:

All the street protocols plus:
道路の項目に加えて：

Frozen/uncompressible chest.
凍結/圧迫できない胸部

Hypothermic patient.
低体温の患者

Putrefaction (rot) is evident.
腐敗が明らかな場合

Hypothermic
低体温

When to stop CPR:
いつCPRを中止するか:

Street:
道路:

Scene becomes unsafe.
現場が安全でなくなった場合

Patient returns to life.
患者が生き返った場合

Rescuer is relieved by equally or more highly trained personnel.
救助者が、同等またはより訓練された他の救助者に交代する場合

Patient is declared dead by an MD, DO, or Medical Examiner.
医師や監察医によって、患者が死亡と認められた場合

Rescuer is unable to continue efforts.
救助者が力尽きた場合

Wilderness:
ウィルダネス:

All of street protocols plus:
路上の項目に加えて：

May stop CPR after 30 continuous minutes without patient exhibiting any signs of life.
CPRを30分間継続しても、患者に蘇生の兆候が現れない場合

EXCEPTION: DO NOT stop CPR if:
例外：CPRを中止しないケース

Patient was victim of:
患者が以下の犠牲となった場合：

A lightning strike: electrocution—may have to provide prolonged ventilations.
落雷にあった場合：感電 – 長時間のCPRを必要とすることがある

A drowning: cold water drowning victims can survive longer durations of submersion.
溺れた場合：冷水で溺れた被害者は、長時間水没していても助かることがある。

AUTOMATED EXTERNAL DEFIBRILLATION
自動体外式除細動器（AED）

Many heart attacks are the result of irregular heartbeats. When cardiac arrest is caused by disorganized ventricular rhythm (ventricular fibrillation), a machine known as a defibrillator can deliver an electrical shock that disrupts or stops this irregular, lethal rhythm, allowing the heart to spontaneously develop an effective rhythm of its own. The sooner a patient in cardiac arrest caused by ventricular fibrillation receives a shock, the greater the chances for survival.

多くの心臓発作は、不整脈の結果として起こる。心室細動により心停止が起こった場合、除細動器は、不整で致命的なリズムを中断または停止し、心臓が自ら効果的な調律ができるように、電気ショックを与える。心室細動により心停止を起こした患者への電気ショックが早いほど、生存の可能性も大きくなる。

Not all cardiac arrests can be helped by a defibrillator. Differing dysrhythmias require differing treatments. Ventricular tachycardia, which is characterized by a very fast lower chamber heart rate, and accounts for less than 10% of pre-hospital cardiac arrests, may also be helped by defibrillation. Neither electromechanical dissociation, which is a very slow heart rate caused by an extremely sick heart muscle, or asystole, where there is no electrical impulse to the heart, can be helped by defibrillation.

すべての心停止が、除細動器によって助かるわけではない。不整脈の種類により、異なる治療が必要となる。心室頻拍（下部の心室の非常に速い心拍で、入院前の心停止の10%以下を占める）は、除細動器により改善されることがある。無脈性電気活動（極度の心筋の疾患による非常に遅い心拍）または心静止（心臓に電気的刺激がない状態）は、除細動器で助けることができない。

Time is of the essence! Six minutes from the moment a person collapses to the moment the defibrillation shock is delivered is considered optimal. Responses are categorized into four segments between the arrest and the first shock, their ideal time components are as follows:

時間が非常に重要である！　最適な条件は、患者が倒れた瞬間から、除細動器による電気ショックが与えられる瞬間までが6分間。心停止から最初の電気ショックまでの応答を4つに区分した場合、理想的な所要時間は以下の通り。

1. EMS (or Emergency Response System) access— from collapse to alerting the EMS system—1 min.

緊急対応システムに通報 – 倒れてからEMSに通報するまで – 1分

2. Dispatch—from EMS receipt of the call to alerting the rescuer—3 min.

出動 – EMSが通報を受けてから救助者に連絡するまで – 3分

3. Response—from the alert to reaching the patient—3 min.

応答 – 連絡を受けて患者の元へ到着するまで – 3分

4. Shock—from reaching the patient to delivering the shock—1.5 min.

電気ショック – 患者の元へ到着してから、電気ショックを与えるまで – 1.5分

If these ideal time goals are met, the survival rate for witnessed cardiac arrest with ventricular fibrillation will improve by 25%.

心停止した所を、誰かが目撃し、心室細動を施し、上記の理想的な時間内で対応ができた場合、生存率は25%UPする。

Public Access Defibrillators (PAD): In an effort to increase survival rates, PAD programs are in place across the country. PADs can be found at airports, malls, sporting events, etc.

Public Access Defibrillators（PAD：公共の場に設置されたAED）：生存率を上げる為に、PADプログラム（公共の場にAEDを設置し、AEDの使い方を含めたCPRのトレーニングを一般市民に普及させる事）は、国内の至る所で取り入れられております。

AEDは、空港、ショッピングモール、スポーツイベント等で利用することができる。

Warnings to be heeded when working with all automated defibrillators:

AEDを使用する際に、注意すべき点：

1. Follow the same precautions that you would for operating any electrical device.

他の電気製品を使用する時と同様 の用心を する。

2. Do not defibrillate a patient who is not in cardiac arrest.

心停止していない患者に除細動を行わない。

3. Do not defibrillate a patient who is in contact with rescuers, bystanders, or others.

救助者や他の人間と接触している患者に除細動を行わない。

4. Do not assess or shock a patient who is being moved or when the defibrillator (or its leads) are being moved.

患者が動かされている時や、除細動器（もしくはコード）が動かされている時に、診断をしたり、ショックを与えたりしない。

5. Do not defibrillate a patient who has an obstructed airway-- the patient who is in respiratory arrest, but not cardiac arrest, does not need defibrillation.

窒息している患者に、除細動を行わない。呼吸停止しているが、心停止のない患者に除細動は必要ない。

6. Do not defibrillate a patient who is in the water.

水中にいる患者に、除細動を行わない。

7. Do not defibrillate a patient who is lying on a metal surface that may transfer the electrical shock to others.

患者が金属の上に横たわっている場合、除細動を行わない。他者に電気ショックが伝わる可能性がある。

8. Do not defibrillate a child who is less than 12 years of age or weighs less than 80 pounds (30 kilograms) unless directed to do so by a physician.

医師の指示なしに、12歳以下または体重30kg未満の子どもに除細動を行わない。

9. All defibrillators are different, but public-access defibrillators are increasingly simple.

全ての除細動器は異なるが、PADは簡単に使用できるようになってきている。

BLS, BLS, BLS...
一次救命処置

1. Perform primary survey to confirm the patient is in cardiac arrest.

患者の心停止を確定するため、第一次診断を行う。

2. Begin CPR. If two or more rescuers are available, one performs CPR while the other prepares and attaches the defibrillator to the patient. If only one person responds, they should follow local protocols.

CPRを開始する。2人以上の救助者がいる場合、1人が患者にAEDを装着する間、他の1人がCPRを実施する。救助者が1人だけの場合は、その地域の規程（プロトコル）に従う。

3. If possible, place the device on the left side of the patient close to the head and work from the left side.

可能であれば、患者の左側、頭部に近い場所にAEDを設置し、左側から作業をする。

4. Bare the patient's chest. If the chest is wet, quickly wipe it dry.

患者の胸部を露出する。胸部が濡れている場合は、素早く拭き取る。

5. Remove the backing from the first pad and place it adhesive side down on the patient's upper right chest. Make sure the adhesive area makes full contact with the skin, and do not press on the mid-section of a pad with a sponge center. The top of the pad should touch the skin over the top of the clavicle while the medial edge is next to the sternum. The pad should not be placed on the sternum.

1枚目のパッドからシートを剥がし、粘着面を患者の胸部右上に貼る。粘着面全面が皮膚に密着するようにし、パッド中央のスポンジ部分を押さないようにする。パッドの上部は、鎖骨上の皮膚に触れるようにし、内側の側辺は、胸骨の横になるように貼る。胸骨の上には貼らない事。

6. Remove the backing from the second pad and

place it on the skin below and left of the left nipple.
2枚目のパッドからシートを剥がし、左の乳
頭の左下に貼る。

7. Tightly connect the lead cables from the AED to the pad following the manufacturer's instructions.
AEDの説明書に従い、AEDに繋がっているケー
ブルをパッドにしっかりとつなぐ。

8. Follow the defibrillator's prompts:
AEDの音声に従う

A. "Stop CPR"—All rescue efforts cease while the AED analyzes.
「CPRをやめてください」－　AEDが解析
している間、CPRを中止する。

B. "Stand back"—All persons must clear themselves of contact with the patient.
「離れてください」　－誰も患者には触
れていない事。

C. "Analyzing rhythm"
「心電図を解析しています」

D. If "Shock advised," you may be instructed to push the shock button.
「電気ショックが必要」な場合は、電気
ショックボタンを押すよう指示がある。

E. After the shock is delivered, immediately restart CPR.
電気ショックを与えたあと、直ちにCPR
を開始する。

F. Perform CPR 5 cycles of 30 compressions to 2 breaths.
胸部圧迫30回＋人工呼吸2回を5セット実
施する。

G. After approximately 2 minutes the AED will tell you to stop CPR so it can analyze the rhythm. It will then either tell you "shock advised" or it will tell you "no shock advised".
約2分後、AEDがCPRを中止する指示を
し、心電図を解析する。AEDより「電気
ショックが必要」か「必要ではない」の
どちらかの指示がある。

H. If a shock is advised, deliver the shock and restart CPR for 5 cycles of 30:2.
「電気ショックが必要」な場合、電気シ
ョックボタンを押し、胸部圧迫30回＋人
工呼吸2回を5セット実施する。

I. If shock is not advised, check pulse. If no pulse, restart CPR.
「電気ショックが必要ない」場合、
脈拍を確認。脈拍がない場合は、CPR
を開始する。

J. Perform CPR 5 cycles of 30 compressions to 2 breaths.
胸部圧迫30回＋人工呼吸2回を5セッ
ト実施する。

K. Continue CPR stopping every 2 minutes to either analyze rhythm again or to check for pulse.
2分毎に中断し、心電図を解析する
か、脈拍を確認しながら、CPRを継続
する。

TROUBLESHOOTING
トラブルシューティング

Most problems, correctable by the rescuer, involve the attachment of pads and/or cables.
救助者によって修正が可能なよくあ
る問題は　パッドとケーブルの装着方法で
ある。

Check to ensure pads are in full contact and cables are tightly connected.
パッドの全面が皮膚に密着していること、
ケーブルが確実につながれていること確認
する。

If pads are not in full contact:
パッドの密着が完全ではない場合:

1. Make sure that the patient's chest is dry and free of anything in contact with its surface.
胸部が濡れていないこと、皮膚の表面に
何も付着してないことを確認する。

2. Remove all dressings and nitro patches on placement site.
すべてのドレッシング（創傷被覆材）と
ニトログリセリンテープを、パッドの貼
用部位から取り除く。

3. Wipe off any nitropaste.
ニトログリセリン軟膏の塗布があれば、
拭き取る。

4. Shave the pad placement area if necessary.
必要に応じて、パッドの貼用部位を剃毛
する。

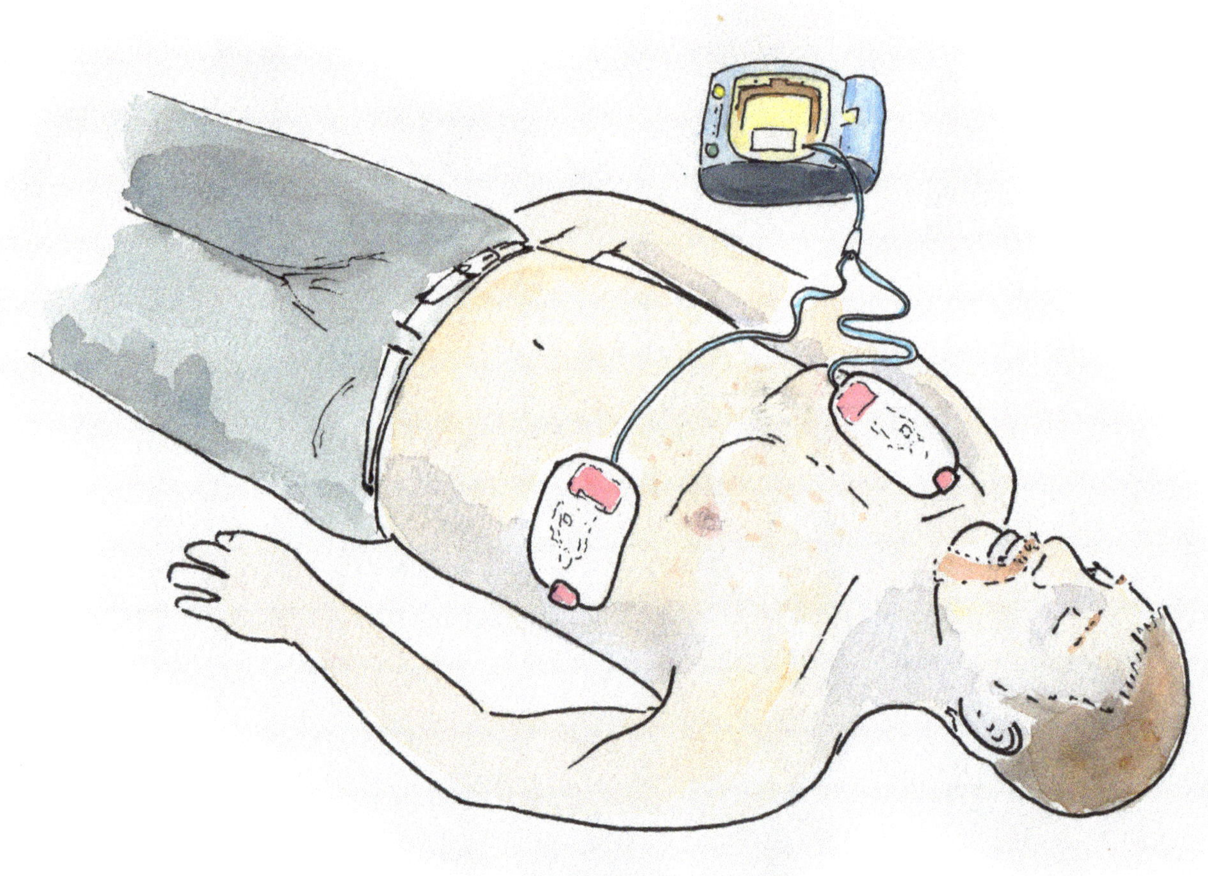

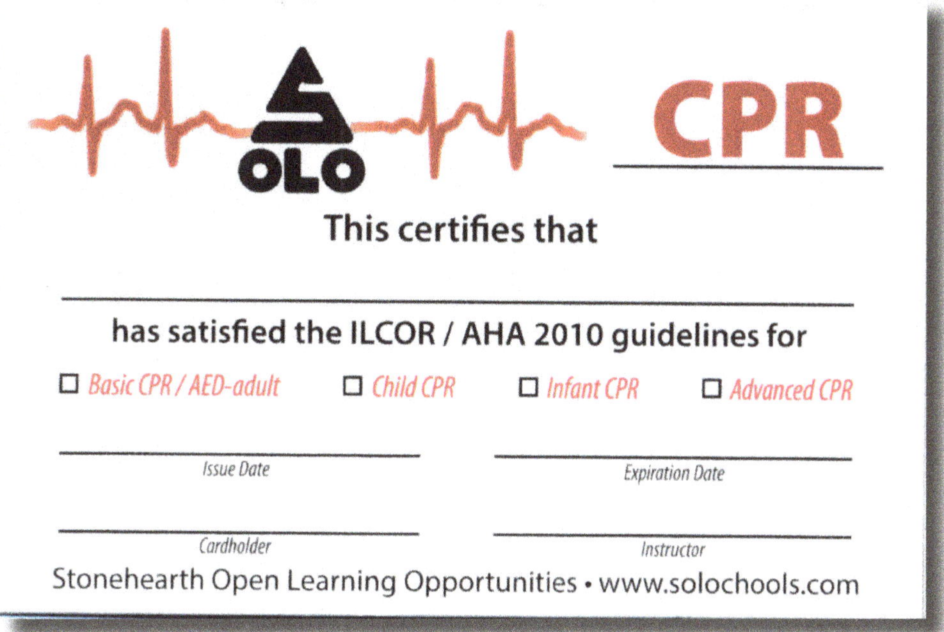

The curriculum for SOLO Basic CPR-AED and Advanced CPR-AED satisfies the requirements for CPR training according to the latest ECC/ILCOR and American Heart Association guidelines. No organization exists that provides a national endorsement or approval for CPR, so each CPR certification provider can develop their own curriculum and implement their own instructional strategies. The SOLO CPR curriculum meets the American Heart recommended guidelines.

SOLOベーシックCPR-AEDと、アドバンスCPR-AEDのカリキュラムは、最新のECC（Emergency Cardiovascular Care：救急心血管治療）/ ILCOR（International Liaison Committee on Resuscitation：国際蘇生連絡協議会）と米国心臓協会のCPRトレーニングの条件を満たしている。CPRについて、全国的な承認を規定している組織は存在せず、それぞれのCPR認定の提供者は、独自のカリキュラムを開発し、独自の指導方略を実施することができる。SOLOのCPRカリキュラムは、米国心臓協会が推薦するガイドラインを満たしている。